THE FELDENKRAIS METHOD

Better Movement, Enhanced Flexibility, And Pain Relief Through Mindful Awareness And Neuroplasticity Techniques

DR. MELISSA STOTLER

Copyright © 2023 by Dr. Melissa Stotler

All rights reserved. Except for brief quotations embodied in critical reviews and certain other noncommercial uses permitted by copyright law, no part of this publication may be reproduced, distributed, or transmitted in any form or by any means, Including photocopying, recording, or other electronic or mechanical methods, without the prior written permission of the publisher.

Disclaimer:

The data in this book, is solely meant to be informative and instructional.

This book is not intended to replace expert medical advice, diagnosis, or care. No medical, health, or other professional services are offered by the author, publisher, or any affiliated parties

Individual outcomes may differ in the practice of these therapies, which entail a variety of approaches and methodologies.

A one-on-one session with a trained or certified healthcare professional is still preferable. It is best to consult a trained healthcare provider before making any decisions regarding your health.

The author of this book is not affiliated with any specific website, product, or organization related to any of these therapies.

All reasonable measures have been taken by the author and publisher to guarantee the authenticity and dependability of the material contained in this book.

Contents

CHAPTER ONE 11
UNDERSTANDING THE FELDENKRAIS METHOD 11
Overview Of The Method..11
The Science Behind Feldenkrais..12
Feldenkrais Vs. Other Somatic Practices......................................14
Core Philosophies Of The Method 15
The Role Of Awareness And Movement......................................16

CHAPTER TWO 19
BASIC CONCEPTS AND TERMINOLOGY 19
Key Terms And Definitions...19
The Importance Of Awareness..21
Functional Integration Vs. Awareness Through Movement 23
The Role Of Movement In Learning 24
Understanding Sensory-Motor Experience..................................26

CHAPTER THREE 29
GETTING STARTED WITH AWARENESS THROUGH MOVEMENT 29
Understanding The Basics...29
Preparing For Your First Session 29
Awareness Through Movement (ATM).......................................30
How To Practice ATM At Home..33
Tips For Effective Practice 34
Common Mistakes To Avoid 35

CHAPTER FOUR 37
FUNCTIONAL INTEGRATION SESSIONS 37

What To Expect In A Functional Integration (FI) Session 37
The Role Of The Practitioner 38
Key Techniques And Approaches 40
How To Prepare For Your Session 41
Understanding Session Outcomes 42

CHAPTER FIVE 45
INCORPORATING FELDENKRAIS INTO DAILY LIFE 45
Applying Feldenkrais Principles To Daily Activities 45
Integrating Feldenkrais With Other Forms Of Exercise 46
Using Feldenkrais For Stress Reduction 47
Enhancing Posture And Movement Efficiency 48
Practical Tips For Daily Practice 49

CHAPTER SIX 51
COMMON CONCERNS AND MISCONCEPTIONS 51
Addressing Common Misunderstandings 51
Clarifying The Role Of Feldenkrais In Rehabilitation 52
How To Choose A Qualified Practitioner 53
Dealing With Skepticism And Misconceptions 54
Understanding The Limitations Of Feldenkrais 55

CHAPTER SEVEN 57
ADVANCED TECHNIQUES AND PRACTICES 57
Exploring Advanced Feldenkrais Techniques 57
When And How To Progress In Your Practice 59
Combining Feldenkrais With Other Modalities 61

Case Studies Of Advanced Practice 63

Safety And Precautions In Advanced Techniques 65

CHAPTER EIGHT 69

RESOURCES AND FURTHER LEARNING 69

Recommended Books And Articles 69

Online Resources And Communities 71

Finding Workshops And Classes 72

Continuing Education In Feldenkrais 73

Connecting With Practitioners And Experts 74

CHAPTER NINE 77

FAQS AND TROUBLESHOOTING 77

Common Questions About The Feldenkrais Method 77

Troubleshooting Common Practice Issues 80

Tips For Overcoming Challenges 82

Finding Support And Guidance 84

How To Track Your Progress And Results 86

ABOUT THIS BOOK

The Feldenkrais Method offers a profound exploration into enhancing human movement and awareness through its unique blend of mindfulness and physical practice. This book serves as an essential guide for understanding and applying this transformative method, which integrates the science of movement with practical techniques for personal development. By delving into the essence of the Feldenkrais Method, readers will uncover the foundational philosophies that set it apart from other somatic practices. The text sheds light on how awareness and movement interplay to foster better body mechanics and self-awareness, offering a comprehensive look at both the theoretical and practical aspects of the method.

Readers will benefit from a detailed introduction to key concepts and terminology, clarifying the critical differences between Functional Integration and Awareness Through Movement. This section emphasizes the importance of understanding sensory-motor experiences and how they contribute to effective learning and movement refinement. Practical advice is provided for beginners, including essential exercises, tips for home practice, and common pitfalls to avoid, ensuring a smooth and productive initiation into Feldenkrais practices.

Functional Integration sessions are explored in depth, offering insights into what to expect during these personalized sessions. Readers will learn about the role of the practitioner, key techniques used, and how to prepare for sessions to maximize their benefits. The book also covers practical advice for incorporating Feldenkrais principles into everyday activities, such as improving posture and movement efficiency, integrating the method with other exercises, and using it for stress reduction.

Addressing common misconceptions and concerns, the book clarifies the role of Feldenkrais in rehabilitation and how to select a qualified practitioner.

Advanced techniques and practices are also discussed, including guidance on when and how to advance in one's practice, and how to combine Feldenkrais with other modalities for enhanced results. The book concludes with a valuable resource section for further learning, offering recommendations for books, articles, workshops, and online communities to support continued growth and understanding of the Feldenkrais Method.

CHAPTER ONE

UNDERSTANDING THE FELDENKRAIS METHOD

Overview Of The Method

The Feldenkrais Method is a therapeutic approach designed to improve movement and function through increased self-awareness. Developed by Moshe Feldenkrais, this method emphasizes gentle, mindful movements to help individuals develop better coordination and ease of movement. At its core, the Feldenkrais Method uses a series of movement lessons, often conducted in either group classes (Awareness Through Movement) or one-on-one sessions (Functional Integration), to encourage learning and improvement in the way people move and function.

In practice, the Feldenkrais Method involves exploring a variety of movements that may seem unusual or unfamiliar. These movements are executed slowly and with a high degree of attention to detail, aiming to identify and release habitual patterns of tension or restriction. The goal is to increase flexibility, reduce discomfort, and enhance overall physical functioning by discovering more efficient ways to move.

The Science Behind Feldenkrais

The Feldenkrais Method is rooted in principles from neurology and motor learning. It leverages the concept of neuroplasticity, the brain's ability to reorganize itself by forming new neural connections throughout life.

By engaging in novel and mindful movements, the method stimulates the brain to create new patterns of movement and coordination. This process helps to break down inefficient movement habits and replace them with more effective ones.

Scientific studies have shown that the Feldenkrais Method can lead to improvements in various physical conditions, including chronic pain, limited range of motion, and functional impairments.

Research indicates that the method can enhance proprioception (the sense of the position and movement of the body), balance, and overall motor control.

This evidence supports the method's effectiveness in helping individuals regain movement capabilities and improve their quality of life.

Feldenkrais Vs. Other Somatic Practices

While the Feldenkrais Method shares similarities with other somatic practices, it also has distinct differences.

Somatic practices, such as Alexander Technique and Rolfing, all aim to improve body awareness and movement. However, the Feldenkrais Method stands out due to its focus on the exploration of movement through a combination of verbal instructions and physical guidance.

Unlike some practices that might focus more on alignment or specific muscle groups, the Feldenkrais Method emphasizes the overall organization of the body in movement. It encourages individuals to explore a wide range of movements and find the most efficient ways to perform everyday tasks. This holistic approach helps practitioners develop greater self-awareness and a deeper understanding of how their movements impact their overall physical and mental well-being.

Core Philosophies Of The Method

The Feldenkrais Method is built on several core philosophies. One of the central tenets is the belief that improved function arises from increased awareness.

By becoming more conscious of how they move, individuals can identify and alter habitual patterns of tension and restriction. This increased awareness leads to a more effective and harmonious way of moving.

Another important philosophy is the idea that learning and change come from a place of ease and exploration rather than force.

The method encourages individuals to approach movement with curiosity and patience, allowing for gradual improvement rather than immediate results.

This non-judgmental approach fosters a safe and supportive environment where individuals can discover their solutions to movement challenges.

The Role Of Awareness And Movement

Awareness is a fundamental component of the Feldenkrais Method. It involves paying close attention to how the body moves and how various movements feel.

By focusing on the sensations and patterns of movement, individuals can become more attuned to their physical processes and identify areas of tension or inefficiency.

Movement in the Feldenkrais Method is approached with a focus on exploration and experimentation.

Rather than performing repetitive exercises, individuals engage in a variety of movements designed to stimulate the brain and body in new ways.

This process helps to uncover more effective and comfortable ways to move, ultimately leading to improved overall function and well-being.

CHAPTER TWO

BASIC CONCEPTS AND TERMINOLOGY

The Feldenkrais Method is a holistic approach to improving physical function and self-awareness through movement. It's named after its founder, Moshe Feldenkrais, who developed the method based on his exploration of the mind-body connection and learning through movement. Understanding the core concepts and terminology can help you grasp how the Feldenkrais Method works and how it can benefit you.

Key Terms And Definitions

Functional Integration (FI): This is a one-on-one hands-on approach where a trained practitioner uses gentle touch and movement to help individuals improve their movement patterns. The goal is to address specific functional issues or areas of discomfort by guiding the person through a series of movements that help them find more efficient and effective ways of moving.

Awareness Through Movement (ATM): In contrast to Functional Integration, Awareness Through Movement involves group classes where individuals follow verbal instructions to explore various movements. These sessions are designed to increase body awareness and improve movement patterns by guiding participants through a series of exercises that highlight different aspects of movement.

Movement Patterns: These are the habitual ways in which we move. They are influenced by our physical habits, emotional states, and past experiences. The Feldenkrais Method aims to help individuals recognize and change inefficient or uncomfortable movement patterns.

Body Schema: This term refers to the internal map or perception we have of our body in space. The Feldenkrais Method helps refine and enhance this body schema, improving overall coordination and movement efficiency.

The Importance Of Awareness

Awareness is central to the Feldenkrais Method. It involves developing a heightened sense of your body's position and movements.

By focusing on how you move and how you feel while moving, you can uncover inefficiencies and habits that may be causing discomfort or limiting your range of motion.

Sensory Awareness: This is the ability to tune into the sensations in your body during movement. Enhanced sensory awareness allows you to detect subtle changes and adjustments, leading to more precise and efficient movements.

Body Awareness: Developing a clear sense of your body's alignment and positioning helps in making conscious adjustments to improve your overall movement quality.

By becoming more aware of how your body moves, you can learn to correct misalignments and reduce tension.

Mind-Body Connection: Awareness in the Feldenkrais Method is not just about physical sensations but also involves connecting these sensations with mental processes.

This connection can lead to a deeper understanding of how movement patterns are linked to emotional and cognitive states.

Functional Integration Vs. Awareness Through Movement

Functional Integration (FI): This approach is highly personalized and tailored to the individual's specific needs.

During a session, the practitioner uses gentle touch and guided movements to help the person become aware of and modify their movement patterns.

FI is particularly useful for addressing specific physical issues or improving overall functional abilities.

Awareness Through Movement (ATM): These are group sessions where participants follow verbal instructions to explore various movements. ATM focuses on self-discovery and developing body awareness through structured exercises.

It is less personalized than FI but offers a broad approach to improving movement and awareness for groups.

Complementary Approaches: While Functional Integration provides individualized attention, Awareness Through Movement offers a more general exploration of movement patterns. Both approaches are complementary and can be used together to enhance overall body awareness and function.

The Role Of Movement In Learning

Movement is a fundamental aspect of learning in the Feldenkrais Method. It is through movement that individuals explore and refine their physical abilities, discover new ways of moving, and integrate these new patterns into their daily lives.

Learning Through Exploration: By engaging in various movement exercises, individuals can discover more efficient ways of performing tasks.

This exploration helps in developing new neural pathways and improving motor skills.

Feedback and Adjustment: Movement provides immediate feedback on how well a particular pattern or technique is working.

By paying attention to this feedback, individuals can make real-time adjustments to enhance their movement quality.

Integration of New Patterns: Learning in the Feldenkrais Method involves integrating new movement patterns into daily activities.

This process helps in making lasting changes to movement habits and improving overall functional abilities.

Understanding Sensory-Motor Experience

Sensory-motor experience refers to the interplay between sensory input and motor responses. In the Feldenkrais Method, this concept is crucial for understanding how movement and sensation are interconnected.

Sensory Feedback: This is the information received through the senses during movement. It helps in assessing how a movement feels and whether it is being executed efficiently.

Motor Responses: These are the physical actions or adjustments made in response to sensory feedback.

The Feldenkrais Method emphasizes the importance of refining motor responses based on sensory input to improve movement efficiency.

Integration of Sensory and Motor Functions: The goal of the Feldenkrais Method is to enhance the integration of sensory and motor functions.

By developing a better understanding of how these functions interact, individuals can improve their overall coordination and movement quality.

CHAPTER THREE

GETTING STARTED WITH AWARENESS THROUGH MOVEMENT

Understanding The Basics

Awareness Through Movement (ATM) is a core component of the Feldenkrais Method. It involves guided movement sequences designed to increase body awareness and improve physical function. To get started, you need to be open to exploring new ways of moving and feeling your body. Approach each session with curiosity and a willingness to listen to your body's feedback.

Preparing For Your First Session

Begin by finding a quiet, comfortable space where you can lie down or sit without distractions. Make sure you have enough room to move freely. It's helpful to have a yoga mat or soft carpet for added comfort. Wear loose, comfortable clothing that allows for unrestricted movement.

Setting an Intention

Before starting, set a clear intention for your practice. This might be as simple as wanting to feel more relaxed or to explore a particular movement pattern. Having a goal helps guide your focus and can enhance the effectiveness of the exercises.

Awareness Through Movement (ATM)

The Concept of ATM

Awareness Through Movement (ATM) exercises involve slow, gentle movements guided by verbal instructions. These exercises are designed to help you develop a heightened sense of how your body moves and functions.

The focus is on quality of movement rather than quantity or intensity.

The Role of the Teacher

Typically, ATM sessions are led by a Feldenkrais practitioner who provides verbal cues to guide you through each movement sequence. The teacher's role is to offer gentle suggestions and adjustments to help you explore and expand your movement possibilities.

Listening to Your Body

As you perform ATM exercises, pay close attention to how your body feels. Notice any areas of tension or discomfort and adjust your movements accordingly. The goal is to find ease and fluidity in your movements, not to push through pain or discomfort.

Basic ATM Exercises for Beginners

Simple Pelvic Tilts

Start by lying on your back with your knees bent and feet flat on the floor. Gently tilt your pelvis forward and backward, feeling the natural arching of your lower back. Move slowly and breathe deeply. This exercise helps increase awareness of your pelvic movements and lower back alignment.

Head Rolls

While lying on your back, gently roll your head from side to side. Focus on the smoothness of the movement and avoid any sudden jerks. This exercise helps release tension in the neck and improves head mobility.

Arm and Leg Coordination

Lie on your back with your arms extended and legs bent. Slowly lift one arm and the opposite leg, then lower them back down. Alternate sides. This exercise enhances coordination and balance between the upper and lower body.

How To Practice ATM At Home

Creating a Comfortable Space

Set up a dedicated area for your ATM practice. Ensure it is quiet, well-lit, and free from distractions. Use a comfortable mat or soft surface to lie on. Having a designated space helps you establish a routine and creates a relaxing environment for your practice.

Following Recorded Sessions

If you don't have access to a live Feldenkrais practitioner, consider using recorded ATM sessions. Many practitioners offer audio or video recordings that you can follow along with at home. Choose sessions that match your experience level and focus on different movement areas.

Maintaining Consistency

For the best results, practice ATM exercises regularly. Aim for short, frequent sessions rather than long, infrequent ones. Consistency helps you develop a deeper awareness of your body and enhances the benefits of the exercises.

Tips For Effective Practice

Stay Present and Mindful

Focus on your body and your movements during each exercise. Avoid getting distracted by external thoughts or concerns. Staying present helps you tune into the subtle sensations and adjustments your body is making.

Move Slowly and Gently

Perform each movement slowly and gently. Rushing through exercises can lead to tension and reduce their effectiveness. Slow movements allow you to explore your body's range of motion and discover areas of tension or restriction.

Breathe Naturally

Remember to breathe naturally throughout your practice. Avoid holding your breath or breathing too deeply. Natural breathing supports relaxation and helps facilitate smooth, effortless movements.

Common Mistakes To Avoid

Overexerting Yourself

Avoid pushing yourself too hard during ATM exercises. The goal is to explore and understand your body's movement patterns, not to achieve a specific physical outcome.

Overexertion can lead to strain and reduce the benefits of the exercises.

Ignoring Discomfort

Pay attention to any discomfort or pain during the exercises. While some mild stretching sensations are normal, sharp or intense pain is a sign that you may be moving too quickly or too forcefully. Adjust your movements as needed and consult a practitioner if discomfort persists.

Skipping the Warm-Up

Always begin with a gentle warm-up to prepare your body for the exercises. Skipping this step can lead to stiffness and limit the effectiveness of your practice. A proper warm-up helps increase blood flow and flexibility, making your practice more comfortable and effective.

CHAPTER FOUR

FUNCTIONAL INTEGRATION SESSIONS

What To Expect In A Functional Integration (FI) Session

Functional Integration (FI) is a core component of the Feldenkrais Method, offering a personalized approach to improving movement and function. During an FI session, you will work one-on-one with a trained practitioner who will guide you through various movements and adjustments tailored to your specific needs.

In a typical session, you will be guided through a series of gentle, hands-on techniques. These movements are designed to help you become more aware of your body and its patterns. You may lie on a table, sit, or stand, depending on the focus of the session.

The practitioner will use their hands to guide your movements and help you explore different ways of moving, aiming to enhance your overall coordination and comfort.

You will not be required to perform any strenuous exercises; instead, the focus is on subtle adjustments and refinements.

Each session is unique and tailored to address your specific concerns, whether they involve chronic pain, mobility issues, or simply a desire to improve your movement efficiency.

The Role Of The Practitioner

The practitioner plays a crucial role in Functional Integration sessions. Their primary function is to observe and respond to your body's movements, guiding you through a process of increased awareness and improved function. They use their hands to provide gentle guidance, helping you explore and understand your movement patterns.

A skilled practitioner will tailor their approach based on your individual needs and goals. They are trained to listen to your body's feedback and adjust their techniques accordingly.

This personalized attention helps ensure that the session addresses your specific issues effectively.

Their expertise in body mechanics and movement allows them to identify and address areas of tension or restriction, facilitating a more fluid and comfortable movement experience.

Key Techniques And Approaches

Functional Integration employs a variety of techniques to enhance movement and function. Some key techniques include:

Gentle Touch: The practitioner uses light, precise touches to guide your movements, helping you develop a better sense of how your body can move more efficiently.

Movement Exploration: Through guided exploration, you will discover new ways of moving that may reduce discomfort or improve your coordination.

Postural Reeducation: The session may involve techniques aimed at improving your posture and alignment, which can help alleviate pain and enhance overall function.

Neuroplasticity Stimulation: The method encourages the brain to form new connections related to movement and sensory perception, fostering lasting improvements in how you move and feel.

These techniques are designed to be gentle and non-invasive, focusing on enhancing your body's natural ability to move comfortably and efficiently.

How To Prepare For Your Session

Preparing for a Functional Integration session involves a few simple steps to ensure you get the most out of your experience:

Wear Comfortable Clothing: Choose loose-fitting, comfortable clothing that allows you to move freely. Avoid restrictive garments that could hinder your movements or cause discomfort.

Arrive Relaxed: Try to arrive at the session in a relaxed state. Take a few moments to breathe deeply and center yourself before the session begins.

Communicate Your Goals: Be prepared to discuss any specific concerns or goals you have with the practitioner. This information will help them tailor the session to meet your needs.

Be Open to Exploration: Approach the session with an open mind and a willingness to explore new movements and sensations. This openness can enhance the effectiveness of the session.

By following these simple preparations, you can help ensure a more effective and enjoyable Functional Integration experience.

Understanding Session Outcomes

The outcomes of a Functional Integration session can vary depending on your individual needs and goals. Generally, you can expect several positive results:

Increased Body Awareness: Many individuals find that they develop a greater awareness of their body and its movements, leading to improved coordination and reduced discomfort.

Improved Movement Efficiency: As you explore and refine your movement patterns, you may notice improvements in how efficiently and comfortably you move.

Enhanced Posture and Alignment: Sessions often lead to better posture and alignment, which can help alleviate pain and improve overall function.

Long-term Benefits: Over time, the insights and improvements gained from Functional Integration can contribute to lasting changes in how you move and feel.

It's important to note that the benefits of Functional Integration may be gradual and cumulative.

Regular sessions can lead to more significant and sustained improvements in your movement and overall well-being.

CHAPTER FIVE

INCORPORATING FELDENKRAIS INTO DAILY LIFE

Applying Feldenkrais Principles To Daily Activities

Incorporating Feldenkrais principles into your daily routine can transform how you experience and manage your body. Start by applying the awareness and movement principles to simple, everyday tasks.

For example, when you're brushing your teeth, pay attention to the way you move your arm and wrist. Notice if there's unnecessary tension or awkwardness in your movements.

By focusing on smooth, efficient movements, you can start to reduce strain and increase comfort.

The key is to bring mindfulness to all your activities—whether it's walking, reaching for something on a high shelf, or sitting at your desk. Each action offers an opportunity to practice the Feldenkrais approach to body awareness and efficiency.

Integrating Feldenkrais With Other Forms Of Exercise

Feldenkrais can be a valuable complement to other forms of exercise, enhancing overall physical well-being. When integrating Feldenkrais with more traditional workouts like running, yoga, or weight training, begin by using Feldenkrais principles to improve body awareness and alignment before starting your exercise routine. For instance, use Feldenkrais techniques to understand and optimize your running stride, which can improve your efficiency and reduce the risk of injury.

Similarly, applying Feldenkrais concepts to yoga poses can help you achieve a deeper and more comfortable stretch. This approach ensures that your movements in various exercises are more mindful and efficient, enhancing the benefits of each activity.

Using Feldenkrais For Stress Reduction

Feldenkrais techniques can also be highly effective for managing stress. Stress often manifests physically through muscle tension and restricted movement. By practicing Feldenkrais awareness and movement exercises, you can learn to release unnecessary tension and promote relaxation. Start with gentle, mindful movements that focus on areas where you feel stress or tightness. Breathing deeply and slowly while performing these movements can help calm your nervous system. Integrating Feldenkrais exercises into your daily routine can help you develop a greater sense of control over your physical responses to stress, leading to a more relaxed and balanced state of mind.

Enhancing Posture And Movement Efficiency

One of the core benefits of Feldenkrais is improving posture and movement efficiency. Start by evaluating your current posture and identifying any habitual patterns that may contribute to discomfort or inefficiency. Feldenkrais exercises focus on re-educating your body to find more natural and comfortable ways of moving. For instance, if you spend long hours sitting at a desk, practice Feldenkrais movements that address common issues such as rounded shoulders or a hunched back. By incorporating these exercises regularly, you can enhance your posture, reduce strain on your muscles, and improve overall movement efficiency in both daily activities and exercise routines.

Practical Tips For Daily Practice

To effectively incorporate Feldenkrais into your daily life, keep the following tips in mind:

Start Small: Begin with short, manageable Feldenkrais sessions and gradually increase the time as you become more comfortable.

Be Consistent: Aim to practice regularly, even if it's just a few minutes each day. Consistency helps reinforce the new movement patterns you're learning.

Stay Mindful: Focus on the quality of your movements rather than the quantity. Pay attention to how your body feels and adjust accordingly.

Use Reminders: Set reminders throughout the day to check in with your body and practice mindful movements, especially during routine activities.

Combine with Daily Tasks: Integrate Feldenkrais exercises into everyday tasks, such as while cooking or cleaning, to make practice more practical and seamless.

By incorporating these practical tips, you can make Feldenkrais a natural and beneficial part of your daily life, leading to improved movement patterns and overall well-being.

CHAPTER SIX

COMMON CONCERNS AND MISCONCEPTIONS

Addressing Common Misunderstandings

The Feldenkrais Method, developed by Moshe Feldenkrais, is often misunderstood in its goals and techniques. One common misconception is that it's merely a form of relaxation or stretching.

While it does involve gentle movements, its purpose is to improve body awareness and movement efficiency through a series of carefully designed exercises.

Feldenkrais focuses on retraining the nervous system to enhance movement patterns and reduce chronic pain.

Another misunderstanding is that Feldenkrais is only for people with physical injuries. In reality, it can benefit anyone looking to improve their overall movement quality, from athletes wanting to optimize performance to individuals seeking better posture and coordination.

Clarifying The Role Of Feldenkrais In Rehabilitation

The Feldenkrais Method plays a valuable role in rehabilitation by addressing the functional movement patterns that contribute to pain and dysfunction.

Unlike traditional rehabilitation methods that might focus on strengthening specific muscles, Feldenkrais aims to retrain the entire movement system. This approach helps individuals discover more efficient and less painful ways to move.

In a rehabilitation context, Feldenkrais can complement other therapies. For instance, if you're undergoing physical therapy for a joint injury, Feldenkrais can help you integrate new movement patterns into your daily activities, which may enhance your overall recovery process.

How To Choose A Qualified Practitioner

Choosing a qualified Feldenkrais practitioner is crucial for achieving the best results. Look for practitioners who have completed an accredited Feldenkrais training program, which typically involves several years of study and supervised practice. They should be certified by a recognized Feldenkrais organization.

A good practitioner should be able to clearly explain their approach and how it will be tailored to your specific needs. It's also helpful if they have experience working with your particular condition or goal. Consider scheduling an initial consultation to discuss your concerns and see if you feel comfortable with their style and methods.

Dealing With Skepticism And Misconceptions

Skepticism about the Feldenkrais Method often stems from a lack of understanding of its principles or visible results.

Some people may question its effectiveness because it doesn't always provide immediate, dramatic changes.

However, Feldenkrais aims for long-term improvement by making subtle adjustments to movement patterns, which can lead to significant benefits over time.

To address skepticism, educate yourself and others about the method's scientific basis and success stories.

Many individuals who have experienced positive changes through Feldenkrais find that sharing their personal stories helps bridge the gap between skepticism and acceptance.

Understanding The Limitations Of Feldenkrais

While the Feldenkrais Method offers numerous benefits, it's important to recognize its limitations.

It may not be suitable for all conditions, especially those requiring immediate medical intervention or surgery.

Additionally, Feldenkrais is not a replacement for conventional medical treatments but rather a complementary approach.

Some people might not experience significant changes, particularly if they have specific, severe conditions or if they do not fully engage with the process.

It's also worth noting that the method requires time and commitment; quick fixes are not typical. Understanding these limitations helps set realistic expectations and fosters a more balanced approach to integrating Feldenkrais into your overall health and wellness plan.

CHAPTER SEVEN

ADVANCED TECHNIQUES AND PRACTICES

Exploring Advanced Feldenkrais Techniques

The Feldenkrais Method, a powerful approach to improving movement and awareness, offers a range of advanced techniques for those looking to deepen their practice. These techniques build on the foundational principles of the Method, which emphasize the importance of awareness and gentle exploration of movement.

Advanced techniques often involve more complex patterns and movements that challenge the nervous system to adapt and learn in new ways. One key aspect is the use of "Functional Integration" (FI) sessions, which are highly individualized. In these sessions, practitioners work one-on-one with a student to address specific movement challenges or goals. The practitioner uses their hands to guide the student's movements, helping them discover more efficient ways to move and improve their overall function.

Another advanced technique is "Awareness Through Movement" (ATM) classes, which involve verbal instructions guiding students through a series of movements. In advanced ATM classes, the movements are often more complex and may involve intricate sequences that require a high level of body awareness and coordination. These classes help students develop a deeper understanding of their movement patterns and improve their ability to move with ease and grace.

Incorporating "Movement Variations" is another advanced practice. This involves exploring different ways to perform the same movement, which helps the nervous system become more flexible and adaptable. By varying movements, practitioners can enhance their ability to respond to different situations and challenges in everyday life.

When And How To Progress In Your Practice

Knowing when and how to progress in your Feldenkrais practice is crucial for continued growth and improvement. Progression in Feldenkrais is not about achieving a certain level but rather about deepening your understanding and refining your skills.

A good time to progress is when you feel comfortable with the basic techniques and have a solid grasp of the foundational principles. You should be able to move with increased awareness and efficiency in your daily activities. If you find that you are consistently achieving your movement goals and experiencing improvement in your overall function, it may be time to explore more advanced techniques.

To progress in your practice, consider working with a Feldenkrais practitioner who specializes in advanced techniques.

They can provide personalized guidance and help you navigate more complex movements and patterns. It's also beneficial to attend advanced ATM classes or workshops to challenge yourself and continue learning.

Another way to progress is to self-explore by integrating advanced techniques into your regular practice. Start by introducing new, more complex movements gradually, paying attention to how your body responds. Keep a journal of your experiences and observations to track your progress and make adjustments as needed.

Combining Feldenkrais With Other Modalities

Integrating Feldenkrais with other modalities can enhance your overall movement practice and address specific needs or goals. The Feldenkrais Method complements various approaches due to its focus on awareness and gentle exploration.

One common combination is Feldenkrais and Yoga. Both methods emphasize body awareness and mindful movement.

Combining them can help you develop greater flexibility and strength while maintaining a high level of body awareness.

For instance, you might use Feldenkrais techniques to explore and refine specific yoga poses, improving your alignment and ease in the poses.

Feldenkrais and Pilates are another effective combination. Pilates focuses on core strength and stability, while Feldenkrais enhances overall movement efficiency and awareness.

Integrating these practices can help you develop a stronger, more balanced body and improve your functional movement patterns.

Incorporating Feldenkrais with Strength Training can also be beneficial. Feldenkrais can help you move more efficiently and safely during strength training exercises, reducing the risk of injury and improving your overall performance.

Using Feldenkrais principles to explore and refine your movements can enhance the effectiveness of your strength training routine.

Case Studies Of Advanced Practice

Case studies of advanced Feldenkrais practice provide valuable insights into the effectiveness and applications of the Method.

These real-life examples illustrate how advanced techniques can address various movement challenges and improve overall quality of life.

One case study involves a dancer who sought Feldenkrais treatment to overcome recurring injuries.

By exploring advanced techniques, including intricate movement patterns and personalized Functional Integration sessions, the dancer was able to enhance their movement efficiency and reduce injury risk. The advanced practice helped the dancer develop greater body awareness and coordination, leading to improved performance and reduced pain.

Another case study features an elderly individual with mobility issues. Through advanced Feldenkrais techniques, including complex Awareness Through Movement sequences, the individual experienced significant improvements in their balance, coordination, and overall mobility.

The advanced practice enabled them to move with greater ease and confidence, enhancing their quality of life.

These case studies highlight the transformative potential of advanced Feldenkrais techniques, demonstrating their ability to address a wide range of movement challenges and improve functional outcomes.

Safety And Precautions In Advanced Techniques

While advanced Feldenkrais techniques offer significant benefits, it is essential to approach them with caution and awareness.

Ensuring safety and taking necessary precautions will help you maximize the benefits while minimizing the risk of injury or discomfort.

First, always consult with a qualified Feldenkrais practitioner before diving into advanced techniques.

A practitioner can assess your current level of practice, provide guidance on appropriate techniques, and ensure that the movements are suitable for your needs and abilities.

Listen to your body and be mindful of any discomfort or pain during practice. Advanced techniques should challenge your movement patterns but not cause strain or injury.

If you experience discomfort, stop and consult with your practitioner to adjust the movements or explore alternative approaches.

It's also important to progress gradually when incorporating advanced techniques. Avoid rushing into complex movements without a solid foundation.

Gradually introduce new techniques and allow time for your body to adapt and integrate the changes.

practice self-awareness and mindfulness during your sessions. Pay close attention to how your body responds to different techniques and movements.

Being aware of your physical and emotional responses will help you make informed decisions about your practice and ensure a safe and effective exploration of advanced Feldenkrais techniques.

68

CHAPTER EIGHT

RESOURCES AND FURTHER LEARNING

Recommended Books And Articles

When diving into the Feldenkrais Method, having a robust list of recommended books and articles can provide invaluable insights.

One seminal book is "Awareness Through Movement: Health Exercises for Personal Growth" by Moshe Feldenkrais himself.

This book introduces the fundamental principles of the Feldenkrais Method and includes practical exercises that you can incorporate into your daily routine.

Another excellent read is "The Elusive Obvious: A New Approach to the Science of Movement and Learning" by the same author, which explores the underlying concepts in a more detailed and theoretical manner.

For those looking to understand how the Feldenkrais Method intersects with other fields, "The Feldenkrais Method: Teaching by Handling" by Ruthy Alon is highly recommended.

It delves into the intricacies of the method and provides a comprehensive overview of the hands-on techniques used in the practice.

Articles in professional journals such as "Feldenkrais Journal" and "Movement & Sport Sciences" also offer cutting-edge research and discussions on the latest developments in the field.

Online Resources And Communities

The internet offers a wealth of resources for learning about the Feldenkrais Method. Websites like the Feldenkrais Guild's official site provide a plethora of information, including introductory articles, detailed explanations of techniques, and listings of certified practitioners. You can also find video demonstrations on platforms like YouTube, where many practitioners and educators share tutorials and workshops.

Online communities, such as forums on Reddit and Facebook groups dedicated to Feldenkrais enthusiasts, are excellent for connecting with others who share your interests. These platforms allow for discussion, advice sharing, and support from fellow learners and experienced practitioners. Websites like "Feldenkrais.com" offer blogs, newsletters, and other digital resources that can help deepen your understanding and practice of the method.

Finding Workshops And Classes

Attending workshops and classes is a practical way to experience the Feldenkrais Method firsthand. Local community centers, wellness centers, and yoga studios often host Feldenkrais workshops. To find these, you can search online for events in your area or visit the Feldenkrais Guild's website, which includes a directory of practitioners and training programs.

Workshops can vary in focus, from introductory sessions for beginners to advanced classes for those with more experience. Participating in these sessions allows you to learn directly from certified practitioners and gain personalized feedback. Many workshops also offer opportunities to connect with other participants, enhancing your learning experience and expanding your network within the Feldenkrais community.

Continuing Education In Feldenkrais

For those looking to further their education in the Feldenkrais Method, continuing education opportunities are plentiful. Advanced training programs and certifications are available for those who wish to deepen their expertise and potentially become practitioners themselves. Institutions such as the Feldenkrais Professional Training Programs offer comprehensive training that covers both theory and practical application.

Continuing education can also be pursued through workshops, seminars, and specialized courses offered by various organizations. These programs often focus on specific aspects of the Feldenkrais Method or explore new research and techniques. Staying updated with the latest developments in the field through ongoing learning ensures that your practice remains current and effective.

Connecting With Practitioners And Experts

Building relationships with experienced practitioners and experts in the Feldenkrais Method can greatly enhance your learning journey. Many practitioners offer private sessions, which provide individualized attention and tailored exercises to address specific needs. You can find practitioners through online directories or by attending local workshops and events.

Networking with experts can also be facilitated through professional organizations and conferences dedicated to the Feldenkrais Method. These events offer opportunities to learn from leading practitioners, engage in discussions about the latest research, and exchange ideas with others in the field. Connecting with practitioners and experts not only helps you improve your practice but also keeps you engaged with the broader Feldenkrais community.

CHAPTER NINE

FAQS AND TROUBLESHOOTING

Common Questions About The Feldenkrais Method

What is the Feldenkrais Method?

The Feldenkrais Method is a system of movement education designed to improve physical function and enhance awareness through gentle, mindful movements. Developed by Moshe Feldenkrais, it focuses on increasing self-awareness and refining motor skills by exploring how we move and learn. The method involves two main approaches: Awareness Through Movement (ATM) classes and Functional Integration (FI) sessions.

How does the Feldenkrais Method work?

The Feldenkrais Method works by engaging the nervous system in a process of learning and adaptation. During ATM classes, practitioners follow verbal instructions to explore various movements, often performed in a slow, deliberate manner. FI sessions involve one-on-one interaction where a practitioner uses gentle touch to guide the individual through movements. Both approaches help to reorganize and optimize movement patterns, leading to improved function and reduced discomfort.

What can I expect during a session?

In an ATM class, you can expect to follow a series of verbal instructions guiding you through specific movements. These classes are typically done in a group setting on mats or chairs. In an FI session, you will work individually with a practitioner who will use gentle touch to help you explore movement patterns. Sessions are designed to be comfortable and accommodating to your needs, with an emphasis on ease and self-discovery.

How long does it take to see results?

The time it takes to see results can vary depending on individual circumstances. Some people notice improvements after just a few sessions, while others may take longer. Consistent practice and engagement with the method generally lead to gradual improvements in movement efficiency, reduced pain, and enhanced overall well-being.

Can the Feldenkrais Method help with specific health conditions?

Yes, the Feldenkrais Method can be beneficial for various health conditions, including chronic pain, injury recovery, and movement disorders.

By improving body awareness and movement patterns, individuals often experience relief from discomfort and enhanced physical function. However, it is always advisable to consult with a healthcare provider before starting any new method, especially if you have specific health concerns.

Troubleshooting Common Practice Issues

Difficulty Following Instructions

If you find it challenging to follow the verbal instructions during an ATM class, try focusing on the general movement rather than getting caught up in the specifics. Remember, the goal is to explore and learn, not to achieve perfection. If needed, ask for clarification from the instructor or use supplemental resources like recordings to reinforce the practice.

Experiencing Discomfort

It is not uncommon to experience some discomfort when beginning the Feldenkrais Method, especially if you are exploring new movements. However, any significant or persistent pain should be addressed immediately. Modify the movements to a level that is comfortable for you and communicate with your practitioner about any discomfort you are experiencing. They can provide guidance and adjust the approach to suit your needs.

Feeling Overwhelmed

Starting a new method can sometimes feel overwhelming. To manage this, break down the practice into smaller, manageable parts. Focus on one aspect of the method at a time and gradually build your confidence. Patience and consistent practice are key. Remember, the learning process is gradual, and progress comes with time.

Struggling with Consistency

Maintaining consistency can be a challenge for many. Establish a regular practice schedule that fits into your daily routine. Set aside specific times for your sessions and create a comfortable practice environment. You may also find it helpful to set small, achievable goals to keep yourself motivated.

Tips For Overcoming Challenges

Start Slowly and Gradually Increase the Complexity

Begin with simple movements and gradually progress to more complex ones. This approach helps you build a strong foundation and reduces the risk of frustration. As you become more comfortable with basic movements, you can slowly incorporate more challenging exercises.

Use Visual and Auditory Aids

Incorporate visual aids, such as diagrams or videos, to help you understand the movements better. Auditory aids, such as recorded instructions or guided sessions, can also enhance your practice by providing additional support and clarity.

Practice Mindfulness and Patience

Approach each session with an open mind and a willingness to explore. Mindfulness and patience are crucial in the Feldenkrais Method. Allow yourself the space to learn and adapt without judgment. Recognize that progress may be gradual and embrace the process of self-discovery.

Seek Feedback and Support

Don't hesitate to seek feedback from instructors or practitioners. They can provide valuable insights and adjustments to enhance your practice.

Additionally, joining a community or finding a practice group can offer support, encouragement, and shared experiences.

Finding Support And Guidance

Consult a Qualified Practitioner

For personalized guidance, consider working with a certified Feldenkrais practitioner. They can provide tailored sessions and address specific needs, helping you navigate any challenges and optimize your practice.

Join a Practice Group or Class

Participating in group classes or workshops can offer additional support and motivation. Being part of a community allows you to share experiences, learn from others, and stay committed to your practice.

Utilize Online Resources

Explore online resources such as instructional videos, webinars, and forums dedicated to the Feldenkrais Method.

These resources can supplement your learning and provide additional perspectives on practice and application.

Seek Professional Advice

If you have specific health concerns or conditions, consult with your healthcare provider or a specialist.

They can offer guidance on how to integrate the Feldenkrais Method into your overall health plan and ensure it complements any other treatments or therapies you may be receiving.

How To Track Your Progress And Results

Keep a Practice Journal

Maintain a journal to track your practice sessions, noting any observations, challenges, and improvements. Regularly recording your experiences can help you identify patterns, monitor progress, and make informed adjustments to your practice.

Set Specific Goals

Establish clear, achievable goals for your Feldenkrais practice. These goals can be related to improving specific movements, reducing discomfort, or enhancing overall awareness. Regularly review and adjust your goals as you progress.

Monitor Physical Changes

Pay attention to any physical changes or improvements in your movement patterns, flexibility, or comfort levels. Tracking these changes can provide tangible evidence of progress and motivate you to continue with the practice.

Seek Feedback from Practitioners

Regularly consult with your Feldenkrais practitioner for feedback on your progress. They can offer professional insights and adjustments to help you achieve your goals and overcome any challenges.

Evaluate Your Overall Well-being

Consider the broader impact of the Feldenkrais Method on your overall well-being, including factors like stress reduction, increased relaxation, and improved daily functioning. Assessing these areas can provide a comprehensive view of the benefits you are experiencing.

www.ingramcontent.com/pod-product-compliance
Lightning Source LLC
Chambersburg PA
CBHW071948210526
45479CB00003B/857